# 25 LANDMARK TRIALS IN CARDIOLOGY

## THIRD EDITION

### Drs. Gabor Gyenes, Craig Butler and Robert Welsh

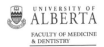
UNIVERSITY OF ALBERTA
FACULTY OF MEDICINE & DENTISTRY

Community Books

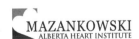
MAZANKOWSKI
ALBERTA HEART INSTITUTE

Design: Brenda Conroy
Printed and bound in Canada by
Hignell Printing, Winnipeg, MB
Published by Community Books
322 Pleasant Point Road, RR1 Lockeport, Nova Scotia, B0T 1L0
phone/fax: (902) 656-2446
email: kathleentudor@eastlink.ca
www.selfpublishingspecialists.com


Copies of this book may be obtained from:
Gabor Gyenes MD PhD, Associate Professor of Cardiology
University of Alberta Hospital, 2C2 Walter Mackenzie
Health Sciences Centre, Edmonton, AB
Canada T6G 2B7
Tel: (780) 407-7929, Fax: (780) 407-6918
gabor.gyenes@albertahealthservices.ca
A mobile version of this book is available
from www.skyscape.com

Library and Archives Canada Cataloguing in Publication

Gyenes, Gabor
25 landmark trials in cardiology / Gabor Gyenes, Craig Butler and Robert
Welsh. — 3rd ed.

Includes bibliographical references.
ISBN 978-1-896496-71-9

1. Heart—Diseases—Treatment—Evaluation—Handbooks, manuals, etc.
2. Clinical trials—Handbooks, manuals, etc. I. Butler, Craig R. (Craig Ronald),
1973- II. Welsh, Robert, 1967- III. Title. IV. Title: Twenty-five landmark trials in
cardiology.

RC683.8.G94 2011     616.1'2060724     C2011-903329-1

# Contents

# Warning/Disclaimer

# Acknowledgements

We are grateful to our families for their love and support and for putting up with our long working hours.

We want to thank Dr. Lisa McKnight for the idea of the book.

We also want to thank Brenda Conroy for the design of the book and both Brenda and Kathleen Tudor for being patient and helpful publishers beyond all expectations.

Publication and distribution of the third edition has been made possible through the generous donation of an unrestricted educational grant from Boehringer Ingelheim Canada.

 Boehringer
Ingelheim

# Preface to the Third Edition

A 56-year-old man presented the prior evening with a troponin positive acute coronary syndrome. After an uneventful night the patient's treatment strategy was being discussed at morning CCU rounds with due attention paid to 'evidenced based medicine.' The residents presented a variety of management strategies with enthusiastic defense of each proposal. "These are all reasonable plans," I interjected, "but what would the evidence have us do?" The response was considerably less enthusiastic. "Well there are only a thousand studies in cardiology, why is it so difficult to remember them all," I commented, trying to sound funny. "Yes there are a thousand studies so why isn't there a book on the most important ones?" asked one thoughtful resident.

The first Edition of this book was thus created in 2005-06 in response to voiced frustrations among junior medicine, cardiology and off-service residents rotating through cardiology as well as non-cardiologist physicians who are overwhelmed by the sheer number of cardiology trials. After repeated requests for references of 'just the important trials' or 'just the trials that changed practice,' Craig and I decided to compile a user-friendly quick-reference guide of the '25 trials' that had the biggest impact on clinical practice across the breadth of cardiovascular medicine. Five years and two Editions later we have altogether distributed and sold almost 20,000 copies of our book — a feat that is in no small part due to our sponsors' ongoing support.

Naturally, the most difficult and contentious part of writing this handbook continues to be the selection of a limited number of landmark studies that really changed the way cardiology is practiced today. With each new addition of "25 landmark trials" we continue to comb through the cardiovascular literature for robust trials that consolidate mature lines of evidence and ultimately persuade us to change practice. Sometimes this means replacing one trial in our book with another, but frequently we try to incorporate new an important trials into our perspective section to support and/or consolidate recommendations. We hope the addition of our editorial remarks facilitate understanding by placing each trial in context and emphasizing important strengths or limitations in the interpretation of trial results — you will be the judge again of how we succeeded.

Further copies can be ordered from gabor.gyenes@albertahealthservices.ca and we always welcome comments and suggestions as well. Digital versions are available at www.skyscape.com. We hope this book will be a useful and relevant companion to you.

*Gabor Gyenes*

# Acronyms and Abbreviations

ACS – acute coronary syndrome

AE – adverse events

(A)MI – (acute) myocardial infarction

ARR   absolute risk reduction

BID – twice daily

CCB – calcium channel blocker

CHD – coronary heart disease

CVD – cardiovascular disease

CI – confidence interval

CK – creatin kinase

CRF – chronic renal failure

c/w – compared with

DM – diabetes mellitus

EF – ejection fraction

EP – endpoint

F/U - follow-up

GP IIb/IIIa – glycoprotein IIb/IIIa antagonists

HF – heart failure

HTN - hypertension

ICD (or AICD) – (automatic) implantable cardioverter-defibrillator

IHD – ischemic heart disease

IVUS – intravascular ultrasonography

JACC – Journal of the American College of Cardiology

LV – left ventricle or left ventricular

LBBB – left bundle branch block

LFT/LE – liver function tests, or liver enzymes

LVD – left ventricular dysfunction

LVEF – left ventricular ejection fraction

Non-STEMI - myocardial infarction without ST-elevation

NS – not significant

NSR – normal sinus rhythm

NSTE ACS – non-ST elevation acute coronary syndrome

NYHA – New York Heart Association (HF classification)

od – once daily

OR – odds ratio

PCI – percutaneous coronary intervention

PVD – peripheral vascular disease

RCT – randomized controlled trial

RR(R) – relative risk (reduction)

SK - Streptokinase

STEMI – ST-elevation myocardial infarction

TC – total cholesterol

tPA – tissue plasminogen activator

UA – unstable angina

ULN – upper limit of normal

# ST-elevation Myocardial Infarction (STEMI) Studies

## GISSI-1

Gruppo Italiano per lo Studio della Streptochinasi Nell'Infarto Miocardico
*Lancet* 1986;327:397-402 and
*Lancet* 1987;330:871-874.

### Study Question
Does streptokinase (SK) reduce morbidity and mortality in myocardial infarction?

### Methods
Multicenter non-blinded randomized trial of 11,806 patients with an acute myocardial infarction (both ST-elevation and ST-depression) within 12 hours of symptoms.
Patients were randomized to 1.5 million units of streptokinase (SK) vs. placebo. In addition all patients received "usual practice" of each recruiting hospital.

### Results
Concomitant Therapy: Heparin iv = 21%, ASA = 13%, Beta blocker = 8%. There were no significant differences between SK and placebo groups with respect to concomitant treatments.

#### 21 day mortality
*SK vs. Placebo:*

| | | | |
|---|---|---|---|
| All patients: | 10.7% vs. 13% | RR 0.81 | p=0.0002 |
| ST depression: | 20.5% vs. 16.3% | | p=NS |
| Killip Class IV: | 69.9% vs. 70.1% | | p=NS |

#### 21 day mortality benefit stratified by time between onset of pain and SK infusion

| | |
|---|---|
| <1 hr RR 0.49 | (95% CI 0.34-0.69, p=0.0001) |
| ≤3 hr RR 0.74 | (95% CI 0.63-0.87, p=0.0005) |
| 3-6 hr RR 0.80 | (95% CI 0.66-0.98, p=0.03) |
| 6-9 hr RR 0.87 | (95% CI 0.64-1.19, p=NS) |
| 9-12 hr RR 1.19 | (95% CI 0.75-1.87, p=NS) |

#### 12 month total mortality
*SK vs. Placebo:*
17.2% vs. 19.0%    RR 0.90 (95% CI 0.84-0.97, p=0.008)

**12 month total mortality benefit stratified by time between onset of pain and SK infusion**

      0-3 h: 15.1% vs. 17.3%     RR 0.89 (95% CI 0.79-1.0, p=0.02)

      3-6 h: 18.3% vs. 21.2%     RR 0.87 (95% CI 0.76-0.99, p=0.02)

      0-1 h: 12.9% vs. 21.2%     RR 0.61 (95% CI 0.47-0.78, p=0.00001)

**Adverse Events**

Major bleeding attributable to SK: 0.3% at 21 days; stroke: 0.2%.

## Conclusion

1.5 million units of SK is a safe and effective treatment for AMI if it can be given within 6 hours of symptom onset.

## Perspective

GISSI-1 was the first large scale study to demonstrate the benefit of fibrinolysis with SK over placebo, demonstrating enhanced short-term and long-term mortality. This trial also underlined the importance of administering reperfusion therapy quickly after symptom onset as evidenced by the fact that the largest mortality reduction was seen in those treated earliest. This trial solidified reperfusion therapy for the treatment of acute ST elevation myocardial infarction and provided the groundwork for further investigations into reperfusion strategies.

The ISIS-2 trial[1] provided the next important step showing the additive benefit of aspirin to SK. This study demonstrated that aspirin alone or SK alone provided similar benefit compared to placebo, but the combination enhanced outcomes in an additive fashion.

1. ISIS-2: *Lancet* 1986;328:57-66.

# GUSTO-1

An International Randomized Trial Comparing Four Thrombolytic Strategies for Acute Myocardial Infarction.
The Global Utilization of Streptokinase and Tissue Plasminogen Activator (t-PA) for Occluded Coronary Arteries Investigators.
*New England Journal of Medicine* 1993;329:673-682.

## Study Question

Multicenter, open label trial to assess 30 day mortality and safety profile of four different thrombolytic protocols in the management of acute STEMI.

## Methods

41,021 patients with STEMI defined as: 20 minutes of chest pain presenting within 6 hours of onset and ST elevation (1 mm in two limb leads, 2 mm in two precordial leads) in two contiguous leads.
Patients were randomized to one of four groups:
1) Streptokinase (SK) + heparin sc, 2) SK + heparin iv, 3) t-PA + heparin iv, 4) t-PA + SK + heparin iv.

## Results

*t-PA vs. Both SK Groups*:

| | | |
|---|---|---|
| 24 hour mortality: | 2.3% vs. 2.9% | (p=0.005) |
| 30 day mortality: | 6.3% vs. 7.3% | (p=0.001) |
| Hemorrhagic stroke: | 0.72% vs. 0.52% | (p=0.03) |
| Allergic reactions: | 1.6% vs. 5.8% | (p<0.001) |

*t-PA vs. SK + t-PA*:

| | | |
|---|---|---|
| 30 day mortality: | 6.3% vs. 7.0% | (p=0.04) |
| Hemorrhagic stroke: | 0.72% vs. 0.94% | (p=0.03) |

*t-PA + SK vs. Both SK Groups*:

| | | |
|---|---|---|
| 30 day mortality: | 7.0% vs. 7.3% | (p=0.352) |
| Hemorrhagic stroke: | 0.94% vs. 0.52% | (p=0.001) |

Absolute mortality benefit for t-PA vs. SK was 1.0% (p=0.001).

Pre-specified subgroup analyses showed t-PA was not better than SK in:
Patients >75 years
Patients with inferior infarctions
Patients presenting >4 hours after symptom onset

## Conclusion

t-PA has a small but important mortality benefit compared to SK in the treatment of acute STEMI.

## Perspective

This trial demonstrated the mortality advantage of the more fibrin-specific t-PA versus SK. This established t-PA as the gold standard reperfusion therapy with a 1% mortality reduction compared to SK albeit at an increased risk of bleeding. Over the next decade intense investigation interrogating alterations of the native t-PA molecule in attempts to create better fibrinolytic agents followed. This has led to the development of single bolus tenecteplase (TNK), which has been shown equivalent to t-PA, and double bolus reteplase (r-PA), as well as other agents that failed to pass the rigours of scientific investigations.

# CLARITY – TIMI 28

Clopidogrel as Adjunctive Reperfusion Therapy – Thrombolysis in Myocardial Infarction 28.

*New England Journal of Medicine* 2005;352:1179-1189.

## Study Question

Does the addition of clopidogrel to thrombolytic therapy improve patency in the infarct-related artery in STEMI?

## Methods

Multicenter international randomized placebo controlled trial that enrolled 3,491 patients, 18-75 years of age with an ST-elevation MI.

Patients were randomized to clopidogrel (300mg loading dose, followed by 75mg once daily) or placebo.

All patients also received: fibrinolysis, aspirin, and heparin. All patients had coronary angiography within 48-192 hours of admission.

## Results

Primary endpoint: composite of an occluded infarct-related artery on angiography or death or recurrent myocardial infarction before angiography.

*Clopidogrel vs. Placebo:*
Primary endpoint:
     15% vs. 21.7%    RR 0.64 (95% CI 0.53-0.76, p<0.001) ARR: 6.7%

*At 30 days:*
CV death/MI/Urgent revascularization:
     11.6% vs. 14.1%   RR 0.80 (95% CI 0.65-0.97, p=0.03).

Major bleeding and intracranial hemorrhage was not different between groups.

## Conclusion

In patients ≤75 years of age with ST-elevation MI, the addition of clopidogrel to the standard fibrinolytic regimen improves the patency rate of the infarct-related artery and reduces ischemic complications significantly.

## Perspective

CLARITY TIMI 28 investigated the impact of additional antiplatelet therapy in combination with standard antithrombotics and fibrinolytics. This followed on the heels of a host of investigations into administration of potent GPIIb/IIIa receptor blockers in conjunction with various fibrinolytic agents and doses, which demonstrated increased risk with no benefit. In contrast, the addition of clopidogrel to aspirin, antithrombotic and standard fibrinolytic therapy demonstrated enhanced patency of the infarct artery with fewer complications prior to an angiogram completed at two to three days post-MI. Although the more standard composite clinical endpoint of death, recurrent MI or urgent revascularization, favoured clopidogrel therapy, the trial was not powered to detect a mortality benefit.

These benefits were achieved without an increased risk of bleeding in this relatively low risk and young population with effectively managed anticoagulation strategy.

The much larger COMMIT-CCS 2 trial[2] conducted in China, tested the addition of clopidogrel without a loading dose (75mg once daily) in 45,852 predominantly STEMI patients. This trial demonstrated a significant though modest mortality reduction consistent with the results of CLARITY TIMI 28.

2. COMMIT-CCS 2 – clopidogrel randomization: *Lancet* 2005;366:1607-21.

# COMMIT – CCS 2

Clopidogrel and Metoprolol in Myocardial Infarction Trial
*Lancet* 2005;366:1622-32.

## Study Question
Do metoprolol and clopidogrel independently reduce adverse outcomes in acute coronary syndromes?

## Methods
Double blind randomized trial with a 2x2 factorial design of 45,852 patients within 24 hours of presentation with a suspected acute MI (93% STEMI or bundle branch block, 7% non-STEMI). Patients were randomized to receive clopidogrel vs. placebo and metoprolol vs. placebo. (The clopidogrel arm is discussed on page 12 with the CLARITY Study.)
Patients were randomized to receive Metoprolol up to 15mg iv, then 200mg po daily or placebo until discharge or up to 4 weeks in hospital.

## Results
Primary endpoints: (1) composite of death, reinfarction, or cardiac arrest; (2) death from any cause.

*Metoprolol vs. Placebo*:

| | |
|---|---|
| Death/MI/Cardiac arrest: | 9.4% vs. 9.9%   (p=0.1) |
| All cause mortality: | OR 0.99 (95% CI 0.92-1.05, p=0.69) |
| Reinfarction: | OR 0.82 (95% CI 0.72-0.92, p=0.001) |
| VF: | OR 0.83 (95% CI 0.75-0.93, p=0.001) |
| Cardiogenic shock*: | OR 1.30 (95% CI 1.19-1.41, p<0.00001) |

*1.1% increased absolute risk for cardiogenic shock was mainly seen within 24 hours of admission.
Metoprolol therapy showed significant harm during days 0-1 and significant benefits thereafter.

## Conclusion
"The use of early $\beta$-blocker therapy in acute MI reduces the risks of reinfarction and ventricular fibrillation, but increases the risk of cardiogenic shock, especially during the first day or so after admission." Consequently, beta blocker therapy at the doses applied in this trial should be given cautiously particularly in the first 24 hours after an AMI.

## Perspective
This beta blocker mega trial has identified the importance of ongoing scientific investigation and the importance of revisiting recommendations that are based on dated data and/or statistical trends. The aggressive dosing strategy

used within this trial is not fully consistent with the current Guidelines' recommendations and it is inconsistent with most physicians' clinical practice. The ongoing judicious use of intravenous and oral beta blockers in appropriate clinical situations remains grounded on scientific evidence and will likely remain incorporated into subsequent clinical guidelines.

# Non-ST-elevation Myocardial Infarction (NSTEMI) Studies

## SYNERGY

Enoxaparin vs. Unfractionated Heparin in High-risk Patients with Non-ST-Segment Elevation Acute Coronary Syndromes Managed with an Intended Early Invasive Strategy.
The Superior Yield of the New Strategy of Enoxaparin, Revascularization and Glycoprotein IIb/IIIa Inhibitors Study.
*JAMA* 2004;292:45-54.

### Study Question
Which heparin has the greatest effect on lowering adverse outcomes in NSTE ACS managed with an early invasive approach?

### Methods
Randomized trial of 10,027 adults with high risk NSTEMI (age >60 yrs, positive cardiac markers or ST segment changes).
Patients were randomized to either enoxaparin 1mg/kg/12 hrs or unfractionated heparin (bolus of 60 U/kg [max. 5000 U] and 12 U/kg/hr [max. 1000 U/h]).
The study protocol dictated mandatory cardiac catheterization (with possible PCI) within 24 hours of admission.

### Results
*Enoxaparin vs. Unfractionated Heparin:*

| | | |
|---|---|---|
| All cause mortality or MI: | 14% vs. 14.5% | (p=NS) |
| Abrupt vessel occlusion: | 1.3% vs. 1.7% | (p=NS) |
| Failed PCI: | 3.6% vs. 3.4% | (p=NS) |
| Emergency CABG: | 0.3% vs. 0.3% | (p=NS) |

**Subgroup analysis:**
75% of patients had been started on a heparin prior to enrollment. Patients without pre-randomization antithrombin therapy and patients who were randomized to the same antithrombin therapy they received pre-enrollment had fewer primary endpoints (death or MI at 30 days) when randomized to enoxaparin therapy (13.5% vs. 14.2% RR=0.82, 95% CI 0.72-0.94) compared to "pretreated and crossover" patients (i.e., started on enoxaparin then randomized to unfractionated heparin iv).

## Primary safety outcome: major bleeding or stroke

*Enoxaparin vs. Unfractionated Heparin:*

TIMI major bleeding:   9.1% vs. 7.6%   (p=0.008)

TIMI minor bleeding:   12.5% vs. 12.3% (p=0.8)

No increase in intracranial hemorrhage, transfusions, or hemodynamic compromise.

## Conclusion

Enoxaparin has similar efficacy to unfractionated heparin, however its convenience is at the expense of a small increase in major bleeding complications.

## Perspective

This trial was designed to confirm the perceived advantage of enoxaparin over unfractionated heparin in a large population of high risk NSTE ACS patients. Despite the prior promising results (e.g., FRISC II[3], ESSENCE[4], TIMI 11B[5], etc.) this mega trial demonstrated no advantage of the low molecular weight heparin enoxaparin in high risk patients with early cardiac catheterization and PCI within 24 hours from admission. Multiple secondary analyses of this trial have been undertaken, demonstrating a host of interesting, albeit hypothesis-generating, points for discussion. Firstly, within this trial a substantial portion of patients were pre-treated with anticoagulation before being randomized. When only those patients who were "anticoagulation-naïve" or on consistent anticoagulation therapy were assessed, the predicted advantage of enoxaparin over unfractionated heparin was demonstrated. Secondly, in countries like Canada, where time to cardiac catheterization was more prolonged, the benefit of enoxaparin was again suggested. Thirdly, there was a strong suggestion that crossing over from one anticoagulant to the other was associated with increased bleeding and ischemic complications.

Although this trial failed to prove the advantage of enoxaparin, it did clarify the importance of consistent anticoagulation with a single agent from the time of admission to hospital through cardiac catheterization, percutaneous coronary intervention, medical stabilization and discharge.

3. FRISC II: *Lancet* 1999;354:708-15.

4. ESSENCE: *N Engl J Med* 1997;337:447-52.

5. TIMI 11B: *Circulation* 1999;100:1593-1601.

# TACTICS-TIMI 18

Comparison of Early Invasive and Conservative Strategies in Patients with Unstable Coronary Syndromes Treated with Glycoprotein IIb/IIIa Inhibitor Tirofiban.

Treat Angina with Aggrastat and Determine Cost of Therapy with an Invasive or Conservative Strategy – Thrombolysis in Myocardial Infarction 18 Study. *New England Journal of Medicine* 2001;344:1879-1887.

## Study Question

Does early invasive therapy reduce adverse outcomes compared to conservative therapy in a population of NSTE ACS patients treated with tirofiban?

## Methods

Randomized controlled trial of 2,220 adults with NSTE ACS who were randomized to early invasive (coronary catheterization <48 hours) or conservative management (coronary catheterization only if recurrent angina or positive non-invasive testing).

All patients received ASA, heparin, and tirofiban.

## Results

*Early Invasive vs. Conservative:*

| | | |
|---|---|---|
| 6 month death/MI/re-hospitalization: | 15.9% vs. 19.4% | (p=0.025) |
| 6 month death or MI: | 7.3% vs. 9.5% | (p<0.05) |

Benefit was seen at 1 week, 30 days and 6 months.

Subgroups:

*Early Invasive vs. Conservative* (Death/MI/re-hospitalization):

| | | |
|---|---|---|
| Positive troponin: | 16.4% vs. 24.5% | (p<0.05) |
| ST segment change: | 16.4% vs. 26.3% | (p<0.05) |
| High risk by TIMI score: | 19.5% vs. 30.6% | (p<0.05) |

## Conclusion

NSTE ACS patients who received coronary catheterization and possible revascularization within 48 hours along with tirofiban treatment had lower rates of death or MI or repeat hospitalization. Subgroup analysis suggests that higher risk patients (elevated cardiac enzymes, ST segment change on EKG, and TIMI risk scores ≥3) receive the most benefit.

## Perspective

There is a long running debate about which NSTEMI patients should have early angiography versus medical management with subsequent angiography if indicated on the basis of clinical deterioration or results of non-invasive testing. TACTICS TIMI 18 is considered by many to be strong evidence for early catheterization in NSTE ACS, in particular for patients with high risk features.

The study was impressive because 51% of the patients on the conservative arm had an angiogram (51% cross-over), 36% had revascularization and despite this the invasive arm (97% angiography and 61% revascularization) still demonstrated significant benefits.

The more recently published ICTUS[6] trial showed no benefit of an early invasive approach in contrast to TACTICS TIMI 18. ISAR-COOL[7], which used aggressive antithrombotic management in both arms with early versus later angiography, was supportive of the results of TACTICS TIMI 18. The logical equipoise between these conflicting data suggests that for patients with truly high risk NSTE ACS ensuring rapid access to cardiac catheterization and appropriate revascularization appears beneficial, as long as this can be achieved within 24-48 hours. Many real life patients do not receive early cardiac catheterization and remain stable in hospital. In these cases a more conservative approach with non-invasive risk stratification guiding invasive therapy is also reasonable.

6. ICTUS: *N Engl J Med* 2005;353:1095-1104.
7. ISAR-COOL: *JAMA* 2003;290:1593-9.

# PLATO

PLATelet inhibition and patient Outcomes (PLATO) trial
*New England Journal of Medicine* 2009 Sep 10;361(11):1045-57.

## Study Question
Is ticagrelor superior to clopidogrel for the prevention of vascular events in patients with unstable angina, NSTEMI, or STEMI?

## Methods
Multicenter, double-blind, randomized trial, comparing ticagrelor (180-mg loading dose, 90 mg twice daily thereafter) and clopidogrel (300-to-600-mg loading dose, 75 mg daily thereafter) for the prevention of cardiovascular events in 18,624 patients admitted to the hospital with an acute coronary syndrome, with or without ST-segment elevation.

## Results
Of patients enrolled 38% had STEMI, 43% NSTEMI and 17% unstable angina. 1 year follow up with time to first event analysis and hierarchical testing of major efficacy endpoints.

Efficacy endpoints:
*Ticagrelor* (n=9,333) vs. *clopidogrel* (n=9,291)

| | |
|---|---|
| CV death + MI + stroke (Primary endpoint): | 9.8% vs. 11.7% (p<0.001) |
| Total death + MI + Stroke: | 10.2% vs. 12.3% p<0.001) |
| CV death + MI + stroke + severe/recurrent ischemia + TIA + arterial thrombosis: | 14.6% vs. 16.7% (p<0.001) |
| MI: | 5.8% vs. 6.9% (p=0.005) |
| CV death: | 4.0% vs. 5.1% (p=0.001) |
| Stroke: | 1.5% vs. 1.3% (p=0.22) |
| Total death: | 4.5% vs. 5.9% (p<0.001) |

Safety endpoints (primary):

| | |
|---|---|
| PLATO major bleeding: | 11.6% vs. 11.2% (p=0.43) |
| TIMI major bleeding: | 7.9% vs. 7.7% (p=0.57) |
| Bleeding requiring red-cell transfusion: | 8.9% vs. 8.9% (p=0.96) |
| Life threatening or fatal bleeding: | 5.8% vs. 5.8% (p=0.70) |

Safety endpoints (secondary):

| | |
|---|---|
| PLATO non-CABG related major bleeding: | 4.5% vs. 3.8% (p=0.03) |
| TIMI non-CABG related major bleeding: | 2.8% vs. 2.2% (p=0.03) |
| PLATO CABG related major bleeding: | 7.4% vs. 7.9% (p=0.32) |
| TIMI CABG related major bleeding: | 5.3% vs. 5.8% (p=0.32) |

Adverse events:

| | | |
|---|---|---|
| Dyspnea (any): | 13.8% vs. 7.8% | (p<0.001) |
| Dyspnea requiring discontinuation: | 0.9% vs. 0.1% | (p<0.001) |
| Ventricular pauses ≥ 3 sec in the first week: | 5.8% vs. 3.6% | (p=0.01) |
| Ventricular pauses ≥ 3 sec at 30 days: | 2.1% vs. 1.2% | (p=0.52) |

## Conclusion

Treatment with ticagrelor as compared to clopidogrel in patients who have an acute coronary syndrome with or without ST-segment elevation, significantly reduced the rate of death from vascular causes, myocardial infarction, or stroke without an increase in the rate of overall major bleeding but with an increase in the rate of non–procedure-related bleeding.

## Perspective

PLATO is the first trial to demonstrate a reduction in CV death in a broad ACS population with ticagrelor compared to established care with clopidogrel. For over a decade dual antiplatelet therapy with ASA and clopidogrel has been the standard of care for patients with ACS.[8,9] This combination has further evidence supporting its use in vascular disease patients in general and in CAD patients that undergo elective PCI.

Ticagrelor is a first in class reversible antiplatelet agent with rapid onset of action, enhanced potency and more consistent effect than clopidogrel that is likely related to ticagrelor's direct action i.e. it is not a prodrug. PLATO confirmed that these properties are associated with enhanced clinical outcomes including a mortality reduction. Although the overall safety profile of ticagrelor was good: it needs to be acknowledged that non-CABG related bleeding was increased and that this agent was associated with the side effects of dyspnea and ventricular pauses. The dyspnea was self limited in the majority of cases and infrequently required drug discontinuation. A dedicated Holter monitoring substudy demonstrated that the ventricular pauses were due to sino-atrial block. The majority (66%) were mostly asymptomatic and did not correlate with any clinically significant adverse events. Significant debate regarding the North American population in the PLATO trial has occurred due to the apparent inconsistency of the results in a predefined regional analysis. It is possible that this apparent difference is due to an interaction with high dose ASA (commonly used in the US) and ticagrelor although a valid potential pathophysiological mechanism has yet to be determined. This issue requires further studies.

The results of PLATO will likely establish ticagrelor and low dose ASA as the new standard dual antiplatelet therapy in the broad population of ACS patients. Clopidogrel will remain the agent of choice in CAD patients undergoing elective PCI and in STEMI patients that receive fibrinolysis since these populations have not been tested with ticagrelor.

8. CURE: *New England Journal of Medicine* 2001;345:494-502.
9. PCI-CURE: *Lancet* 2001;358:527-533.

# Atherosclerosis/Chronic Stable Angina

## COURAGE

Optimal Medical Therapy with or without PCI for Stable Coronary Disease. The Clinical Outcomes Utilizing Revascularization and Aggressive Drug Evaluation Trial.
*New England Journal of Medicine* 2007;356:1503-16.

### Study Question
Does PCI improve hard outcomes over and above optimal medical therapy (OMT) alone in patients with chronic stable angina?

### Methods
Randomized trial of 2287 patients with stable angina, objective evidence of ischemia and a significant stenosis in at least one coronary artery that was amenable to PCI. Patients were randomized to either PCI + OMT (PCI group) or OMT.

The primary outcome was death from any cause and nonfatal MI during a median follow-up period of 4.6 years.

PCI was performed with the intent of full revascularization.

Medical management: aspirin or clopidogrel; lipid-lowering by simvastatin + ezetimibe to achieve an LDL-cholesterol of 1.55-2.2 mmol/l; secondary targets: HDL-cholesterol to be raised over 1.03 mmol/l and TG lowered below 1.69 mmol/L; anti-ischemic therapy: metoprolol, amlodipine, isosorbide mononitrate; lisinopril or losartan for HTN. Patients received smoking cessation and weight loss counseling.

### Results
35,539 patients were screened, 3071 met eligibility criteria, 2287 were randomized.

Median time from first angina to randomization was 5 months (58% Class II or III).

Two-thirds of patients had multiple perfusion defects on stress imaging and multivessel CAD. Significantly more patients had proximal LAD disease in the OMT group.

**PCI:** 94% received a stent (41% >1 stent) with the majority being bare metal (95%). The majority of patients (89%) had "clinical success" i.e. all lesions were successfully dilated without in-hospital complications.

**OMT:** The mean baseline LDL-level was 2.5 mmol/L and at 5 years 70% of subjects had an LDL < 2.2 mmol/L with a median of 1.84 mmol/L; 93% of patients were taking a statin.

The target BP of 130 mmHg systolic and 85 mmHg diastolic were achieved by 65% and 94%, respectively.

$HbA_1c$ of 7.0% was achieved in 45% of the diabetic patients.

Smoking cessation at 5 years was achieved in 6% of PCI vs. 3% of OMT patients.

BMI did not change significantly in either group.

### Incidence of Major Outcomes

*PCI vs. OMT:*

Death and non-fatal MI:

| | |
|---|---|
| 19.0% vs. 18.5% | HR 1.05 (95% CI 0.87-1.27, p=0.62) |

Death, MI and stroke:

| | |
|---|---|
| 20.0% vs. 19.5% | HR 1.05 (95% CI 0.87-1.27, p=0.62) |

Death:

| | |
|---|---|
| 7.6% vs. 8.3% | HR 0.87 (95% CI 0.65-1.16, p=0.38) |

Revascularisation:

| | |
|---|---|
| 21.1% vs. 32.6% | HR 0.60 (95% CI 0.51-0.71, p<0.001) |

| Angina free patients (%) | PCI | vs. | OMT | p-value |
|---|---|---|---|---|
| At baseline: | 12 | | 13 | NS |
| At 1 year: | 66 | | 58 | <0.001 |
| At 3 years: | 72 | | 67 | 0.02 |
| At 5 years: | 74 | | 72 | NS |

## Conclusion

In patients with stable coronary artery disease PCI added to optimal medical therapy did not reduce the risk of death or myocardial infarction. PCI improved angina faster and more efficiently but this difference was only seen for the first 3 years of follow-up.

## Perspective

It has been assumed, based on old evidence, that patients with provokable ischemia and stable coronary artery disease with or without angina would experience a reduction of hard outcomes from percutaneous revascularization. This assumption has led us to aggressively search for any ischemia followed by an attempt at revascularization. Many patients also received "preventive PCIs" of previously asymptomatic severe coronary artery stenosis under the same umbrella of assumptions. The older studies showing advantage of PCI over medical therapy are likely no longer relevant given the impressive improvement in medical therapy in the last decade. In addition, treatment targets have become more aggressive particularly with regard to blood pressure targets and lipid-lowering with statins. The majority of COURAGE patients in fact achieved contemporary blood pressure and lipid targets even though Guidelines at the time of recruitment were less aggressive. This study demonstrates that we need to change our current practice, and consider aggressive OMT as a safe and effective initial strategy in these moderate risk patients. PCI remains a very effective tool in treating resistant angina. Nevertheless, it has to be accepted both by patient and doctor that these patients remain at increased risk for recurrent hard events (> 4%/year in this study) and this risk cannot be changed by successfully dilating the currently worst-looking lesions. Of note, this does not seem to be the case with unstable coronary plaques found in acute coronary syndromes where PCI has been conclusively shown to reduce hard outcomes (see e.g. TACTICS-TIMI 18 on page 17).

A few important points however, are worth further discussion: The generalizability of the findings has been called in question as less than 10% of those screened were deemed eligible for the study. The main reason given by the investigators is that the majority of the ineligibles were too low-risk.

Patients enrolled in the study were almost exclusively white males (85%) and PCI has been suggested (even in this study) to be potentially more successful in women than in men.

The quality of PCI delivered in the study was criticized by some as suboptimal. Only 89% of patients initially randomized to PCI achieved "clinical success" as defined above. This may have been due to the need for treating bifurcation lesions involving side-branches which in fact would fairly reflect "real-life" multivessel PCI. The current, more frequent use of drug-eluting stents (DES) could have decreased the risk of in-stent restenosis and secondary events. However, DES have not been shown to decrease the risk of death and MI when compared to bare metal stents.

Medical therapy was unrealistically optimal compared with that in real life because patient compliance was significantly increased by regular phone-calls from study nurses. No prior study has achieved 90% statin use in both arms at 5 years. At the same time this study proves that these results are not impossible to achieve if we can improve compliance. Maybe our focus should shift in this patient group with chronic stable angina to try and improve adherence to medical management.

The COURAGE results are consistent with the majority of prior evidence that despite being an effective treatment for anginal symptoms, PCI in chronic stable angina does not reduce the risk of hard outcomes and it should not be expected to do so in even lower risk patients either.

# Atherosclerosis/Epidemiology

## FRAMINGHAM STUDY

Framingham risk score reference: *JAMA* 2001;285:2486.
Recent Framingham references: *Int J Cardiol* 2005;104:228;
*Circulation* 2005;112:1113-20; *Circulation* 2005;112:969-75;
*Diabetologia* 2005;48:1492-5; and *Circulation* 2008;117:743-53.
Framingham Offspring publications: *Am J Epidemiol* 2005;162:644-53;
*Clin Cardiol* 2005;28:247-51; *Am J Cardiol* 2004;94:1561-3,
*Circulation* 2004;110:380-5, and *JAMA 2005;294:3117-23*.

### Study Question

Are there risk factors for atherosclerosis? What is the natural history of
atherosclerotic vascular disease?

### Methods

This is an ongoing epidemiological study of a small town called Framingham,
Massachusetts, which started in 1948 and is sponsored by the National Heart
Lung and Blood Institute. Originally, it enrolled 5,209 healthy residents
between 30 and 60 years of age.
The Framingham Offspring study was initiated in 1971, and it recruited 5,124
children (and their spouses) of the original cohort.

### Results

The study resulted in more than a 1,000 papers.
Some of its key findings regarding cardiovascular risk factors such as age,
gender, blood pressure, and smoking were incorporated in the Framingham
risk score, which is widely used to assess an individual's cardiovascular risks
in the following 10 years. Family history of cardiovascular disease was not
incorporated in this score; however, it was addressed by the Framingham
Offspring study that showed:

Sibling CV disease (brothers <55, sisters <65 yr):
  Age- and sex-adjusted   OR 1.55      (95% CI 1.19-2.03)
  Risk factor-adjusted    OR 1.45      (95% CI 1.10-1.91).
Adjusted for sibling and parental CVD with both parents included in the study:
  OR for sibling          CVD 1.99     (95% CI 1.32-3.00)
  OR for parental         CVD 1.45     (95% CI 1.02-2.05).

## Perspective

This study coined the term "risk factors" and helped establish the connection between atherosclerosis and high total and LDL-cholesterol levels, as well as low HDL-cholesterol levels, smoking, hypertension and diabetes mellitus.

Before the Framingham Study atherosclerosis was thought to be a part of normal aging and as such was considered non-modifiable. It was also the first major cardiovascular study to recruit female participants.

The Framingham Offspring study illustrated that a positive family history for coronary disease was not as significant as was previously thought.

The most frequently mentioned criticism of the study is that it almost exclusively investigated a Caucasian population. Therefore, recently, 500 members of Framingham's minority community have been recruited to participate in the Omni Study.

INTERHEART[10] is another large epidemiologic study that evaluated the attributable risk of cardiovascular risk factors in a multi-country, multi-ethnicity, and multi-sociodemographic population. Their findings increase the generalizability of the conclusions drawn by the Framingham studies by showing that conventional risk factors account for most of the risk for myocardial infarction in disparate populations across the globe. However, a recent INTERHEART[11] publication demonstrated that a family history of coronary disease is a significant and independent risk factor for myocardial infarction in a global population just as it is for the Framingham offspring population. A positive family history in one parent (OR: 1.7) or two parents (OR: 2.3) significantly predicted myocardial infarction even after controlling for nine traditional risk factors.

10. INTERHEART: *Lancet* 2004;364:937-952.

11. An INTERHEART Substudy: Parental History and MI Risk Across the World. *JACC* 2011;57:619-627.

# Atherosclerosis/Cardiovascular Protection

## HOPE/MICROHOPE

Effects of an ACE Inhibitor, Ramipril, on Cardiovascular Events in High-risk Patients.

The Heart Outcomes Prevention Study

*New England Journal of Medicine* 2000;342:145-153, and

*New England Journal of Medicine* 2000;342:154-160.

## MICRO-HOPE

*Lancet* 2000;355:253-259.

### Study Question

Does the ACE inhibitor ramipril reduce cardiovascular events in high risk patients with normal ejection fractions?

### Methods

Randomized double blind trial of 9,297 high risk patients over the age of 55 with an LV ejection fraction >40%. High risk was defined as one of the following: 1) History of CHD 2) History of stroke 3) History of PVD 4) DM + 1 other CV risk factor.

Patients were randomized according to a 2 x 2 factorial design comparing ramipril 10mg vs. placebo as well as vitamin E vs. placebo. Patients were followed for 5-years.

MICRO-HOPE, a sub-study focusing on 3,577 diabetic patients treated with ramipril vs. placebo with respect to macro and renovascular outcomes. It was stopped early (4.5 years) due to highly significant and wide ranging benefit of ramipril treatment.

### Results

Baseline BP (139/79 mmHg) was not different between groups.
Ramipril lowered BP by 3/2 mmHg compared to placebo.

Primary endpoint: composite of CV death, MI or stroke.
*Ramipril vs. Placebo:*

| | | |
|---|---|---|
| Death/MI/stroke: | 14% vs. 17.8% | (p<0.001) |
| Overall mortality: | 10.4% vs. 12.2% | (p<0.005) |
| Myocardial infarction: | 9.9% vs. 12.3% | (p<0.001) |
| Stroke: | 3.4% vs. 4.9% | (p<0.001) |
| New diagnosis of diabetes: | 3.6% vs. 5.4% | (p<0.001) |

Benefits were seen after 1 year of treatment.

MICRO-HOPE

*Ramipril vs. Placebo*:

| | | |
|---|---|---|
| Death/MI/stroke: | 15.3% vs. 19.8% | (p=0.0004) |
| Cardiovascular mortality: | 6.2% vs. 9.7% | (p=0.0001) |
| MI: | 10.2% vs. 12.9% | (p=0.01) |
| CHF: | 11% vs. 13.3% | (p=0.02) |
| Stroke: | 4.2% vs. 6.1% | (p=0.007) |
| Overt nephropathy: | 6.5% vs. 8.4% | (p=0.03) |

## Conclusion

"Ramipril significantly reduces the rates of death, MI, and stroke in a broad range of high-risk patients who are not known to have a low LV ejection fraction or heart failure." Vitamin E on the other hand did not affect cardiovascular outcomes in this patient population.

## Perspective

This was the first trial to show the benefit of ACE inhibitors in patients with normal ejection fraction. HOPE demonstrated an impressive reduction in microvascular and macrovascular events with ramipril in all of the subgroups. After the release of HOPE ramipril, and ACE inhibitors in general, quickly became routine therapy for patients with vascular disease, and the term "vascular protection" was coined based largely on this study's outcome.

Some critics claim that it was the BP reduction in the ramipril group, not the drug itself that accounted for the observed benefits. However, previous hypertension trials required much larger reductions in blood pressure to achieve a similar magnitude of effect.

Despite the benefits of ramipril within the HOPE trial population, recent trials have brought into question the general utilization of ACE inhibitors in patients with atherosclerotic disease. The EUROPA[13] trial randomized patients with stable coronary artery disease to perindopril or placebo. This study showed a significant benefit in the combined endpoint of cardiac morbidity and mortality but overall mortality was not significantly improved by the ACE inhibitor. The third, similarly designed trial, PEACE[14] surprisingly failed to show prevention of macrovascular events with ACE inhibitor treatment. When the baseline characteristics of HOPE, EUROPA and PEACE were compared it was apparent that the more recent trials had a higher prevalence of revascularization procedures a lower proportion of diabetics and a greater proportion of patients received lipid lowering therapy. The net effect was that the placebo group in the PEACE trial had cardiovascular event rates that were so low that they approached that of the general population, making it very difficult to show further significant benefits.

Results of PEACE and IMAGINE[12] – another neutral ACE inhibitor trial – have significantly tempered the enthusiasm for ACE inhibitors that the HOPE results had generated. The two neutral trials have illustrated that ACE-inhibitor treatment on top of other treatment modalities such as complete revascularization and aggressive lipid-lowering currently may be of less benefit than prior studies had indicated. However, there remains a broad spectrum of patients in whom ACE-inhibition provides significant benefit such as patients with HF/LVD, AMI, DM, HTN, CRF and in some patients, without any of the above, vascular disease.

12. IMAGINE: *Circulation* 2008;117:24-31.
13. EUROPA: *Lancet* 2003;362:782-788.
14. PEACE: *N Engl J Med* 2004;351:2058-68.

# ONTARGET

Telmisartan, Ramipril, or Both in Patients at High Risk for Vascular Events
*New England Journal of Medicine* 2008;358:1547-59.

# TRANSCEND

*Lancet* 2008;372:1174-83.

## Study Question
**OT:** Does the angiotensin receptor blocker telmisartan or its combination with ramipril reduce cardiovascular risks in high risk vascular patients as well as ramipril alone?
**T:** Does telmisartan provide vascular protection to ACEI-intolerant patients?

## Methods
**OT:** Randomized double-blind non-inferiority trial of 25,620 patients with documented vascular disease randomized into one of three groups: ramipril 10mg, telmisartan 80mg, or the combination. There was a 3-week run-in period before randomization in both studies.
Primary composite outcome: cardiovascular death (CVD), MI, stroke, and hospitalization for heart failure (HHF).
Median follow-up was 4 years and 8 months.
**T:** 5926 patients with vascular disease or DM and end-organ damage were randomized to telmisartan 80mg daily or placebo. Outcomes were similar to those of the OT. Median follow-up was 56 months.

## Results
**OT:** Baseline BP was 142/82 mmHg before the run-in period. At 6 weeks the mean BP reduction was 6.4/4.3, 7.4/5.0, 9.8/6.3 mmHg in the respective groups. Throughout the study telmisartan and the combination lowered BP by 0.9/0.6 mmHg, and 2.4/1.4 mmHg, respectively, compared to ramipril.

Primary endpoint:
*Ramipril vs. Telmisartan vs. Combination:*

| | | |
|---|---|---|
| CVD/MI/stroke/HHF: | 16.5% vs. 16.7% vs. 16.3% | |
| T vs. R − RR: 1.01 (95% CI 0.94-1.09) | | |
| C vs. R − RR: 0.99 (95% CI 0.92-1.07) | | |
| Overall mortality: | 11.8% vs. 11.6% vs. 12.5% | NS |
| Myocardial infarction: | 4.8% vs. 5.2% vs. 5.2% | NS |
| Stroke: | 4.7 % vs. 4.3% vs. 4.4% | NS |
| HHF: | 4.1% vs. 4.6% vs. 3.9% | NS |

Adverse Events

*Ramipril vs. Telmisartan vs. Combination:*

K > 5.5 mmol/L:

   283 vs. 287 vs. 480 patients (p<0.001)

Renal impairment:

   10.2% vs. 10.6% vs. 13.5%; C vs. R – RR 1.33 (95% CI 1.22-1.44) p<0.001

Drug discontinuation due to cough:

   4.2% vs. 1.1% vs. 4.6%       T vs. R – RR 0.26 p<0.001

Drug discontinuation due to angioedema:

   0.3% vs. 0.1% vs. 0.2%       T vs. R – RR 0.4 p<0.01

### TRANSCEND

*Telmisartan vs. Placebo:*

CV Death/MI/stroke/HHF:

        15.7% vs. 17.0% (HR: 0.92; 95% CI 0.81-1.05, p=0.216)

CV death/MI/stroke (HOPE outcome):

        13.0% vs. 14.8% (HR: 0.87; 95% CI 0.76-1.0 p=0.048 unadjusted)

### Adverse Events

Permanent discontinuation of study medication:

     *Telmisartan vs. Placebo:* 21.6% vs. 23.8% p=0.055

## Conclusion

**OT:** Telmisartan was neither inferior nor superior to ramipril in preventing hard outcomes in patients at high-risk for vascular events. The combination was associated with an increased risk of adverse events without improving outcomes.

**T:** Although telmisartan was well tolerated it did not significantly improve the primary combined endpoint. It modestly reduced the secondary endpoint of CV death, MI and stroke.

## Perspective

The ONTARGET Study helps put an end to a decade-long debate about the relative risks and benefits of ARBs vs. ACE inhibitors. Its results unequivocally refuted the suggestion that ARBs are associated with an increased risk of CV mortality or morbidity and it also extinguished the hopes of those who believed in the superiority of ARBs over ACE inhibitors on a theoretical basis.

The weight of evidence regarding ACEIs and ARBs suggest that the two drug classes are effectively interchangeable. In addition, the therapeutic benefits of ACEIs and ARBs are most likely class effects, however it is important to remember that the greatest evidence always lies with the specific drug and dosage tested in clinical trials. It is likely that cardiologists will continue to prescribe ACEIs as a first line choice, however the superior tolerability of the

ARBs will likely result in their increased use particularly for the treatment of hypertension.

ONTARGET also argues strongly against using ACEIs and ARBs in combination for non-heart failure indications. This is consistent with previous findings in VALIANT[15] which was the second largest ACEI/ARB trial. ACEI/ARB combination therapy has shown some benefit in the treatment of CHF in the CHARM-Added study (see page 45). However, this study population had recurrent symptomatic CHF despite appropriate ACEI therapy before the ARB, Candesartan was added, whereas in ONTARGET and VALIANT the combination was started simultaneously.

There may also be a role for the combination in refractory hypertension although this was not tested in either of the above-mentioned studies. Close follow-up of electrolytes and renal function is warranted in these patients who are at increased risk for worsening renal failure.

The surprisingly modest results of the TRANSCEND Study may reflect the fact that it was underpowered or that the follow-up was not long enough. It also may reflect on the changed environment compared to that of the HOPE study in which the placebo group had a 3% higher event rate. However, the excellent tolerability of telmisartan is good news for patients who have an indication to take an ACE inhibitor but can't tolerate it. See also the discussion of the HOPE, EUROPA and PEACE trials on page 26.

15. VALIANT: *N Engl J Med* 2003;349:1893-1906.

# Lipid Studies

## 4S

Randomized Trial of Cholesterol Lowering in 4,444 Patients with Coronary Heart Disease: The Scandinavian Simvastatin Survival Study
*Lancet* 1994;344:1383-1389, and
*Lancet* 1995;345:1274-1275.

### Study Question
Does simvastatin reduce mortality in patients with coronary disease and hyperlipidemia?

### Methods
Double blind randomized placebo controlled trial of 4,444 patients with elevated cholesterol (total cholesterol 5.5-8.0 mmol/L) and a history of coronary disease defined as angina or prior MI.
Patients were randomized to simvastatin (S) 20mg (titrated to achieve a TC<5.2 mmol/L) vs. placebo (Pl).
Median follow up was 5.4 years.

### Results
Simvastatin dose: 20mg (63%), 40mg (37%)
Simvastatin reduced LDL by 38% and increased HDL by 8%.

*Simvastatin vs. Placebo:*
All cause mortality:
      8.2% vs. 11.5%  RR 0.70 (95% CI 0.58-0.85, p=0.0003)
Coronary mortality:
      5% vs. 8.5%    RR 0.58 (95% CI 0.46-0.73)
Non-CV mortality:      NS
≥1 major coronary event:
      19% vs. 28%    RR 0.66 (95% CI 0.59-0.75, p<0.00001)

Mortality benefit was evident after 1.5 years of treatment.
Reduction in coronary events was evident after 1 year.
Benefits were the same regardless of baseline cholesterol levels.

#### Adverse Events
*Simvastatin vs. Placebo:*
Rhabdomyolysis: 1 vs. 0 case
CK elevation >10x ULN: 6 vs. 1 cases

## Conclusion

Long-term reduction of cholesterol levels with simvastatin is safe and effective in achieving a significant reduction in both coronary morbidity and mortality.

## Perspective

Prior to the 4S trial there was no conclusive evidence that reducing cholesterol levels would reduce cardiovascular mortality. The results of the 4S trial established LDL lowering as one of the cornerstones of cardiovascular disease prevention. By reducing LDL cholesterol levels by 38%, simvastatin lowered all cause mortality by an impressive 30%. There are very few therapies in cardiology that are this effective at lowering mortality. This trial provided the groundwork for a host of trials that tested the impact of lipid reduction across a broad spectrum of patient populations with CVD.

# HPS

MRC/BHF Heart Protection Study of Cholesterol Lowering with Simvastatin in 20,536 High-risk Individuals: A Randomized Placebo Controlled Trial
*Lancet* 2002;360:7-22, and
*Lancet* 2003;361:2005-16 (Diabetic sub-study).

## Study Question
Does simvastatin, vitamins or both prevent cardiovascular outcomes in individuals with relatively normal cholesterol levels, but with documented vascular disease or multiple CV risk factors?

## Methods
Double blind randomized placebo controlled trial with a 2 x 2 factorial design of 20,536 adults with stable CAD, PVD, or Type II DM.
Patients were randomized according to a 2 x 2 factorial design to:
>    simvastatin 40mg or placebo, and
>    vitamins (vit E 600mg, vit C 250mg, $\beta$-carotene 20mg) or placebo.
Five years of follow up.

## Results
### Incidence of major outcomes
*Simvastatin vs. Placebo:*

| | |
|---|---|
| All-cause mortality: | 12.9% vs. 14.7% (p=0.0003) |
| Cardiac mortality: | 5.7% vs. 6.9%  (p=0.0005) |
| Nonfatal MI or CV death: | 8.7% vs. 11.8%  (p=0.0001) |
| Stroke: | 4.3% vs. 5.7%  (p=0.0001) |
| Any vascular event: | 19.8% vs. 25.2% (p=0.0001) |

The benefits of simvastatin were similar irrespective of age, gender, or baseline cholesterol. Benefit was even seen in those with an LDL-C of less than 3.0 mmol/L.

### Adverse events
*Simvastatin vs. Placebo:*

| | |
|---|---|
| Risk of myopathy: | 0.01% per year |
| Muscle symptoms: | 0.5% vs. 0.5%  (p=NS) |
| Liver enzyme elevations (>4 ULN): | 0.09% vs. 0.04% (p=NS) |
| Malignancy: | 7.9% vs. 7.8%  (p=NS) |

Diabetic patients had a more pronounced benefit from simvastatin.
Vitamins did not significantly lower the rate of cardiovascular events.

## Conclusion

Simvastatin 40mg reduced mortality and major vascular events in high risk patients irrespective of their initial cholesterol levels.

## Perspective

This was the first study to suggest that lowering LDL and total cholesterol levels with statin therapy should be a treatment goal for every patient at high risk for cardiovascular events irrespective of their baseline cholesterol levels. This concept ran contrary to the prevailing guidelines at the time. This trial showed that treating cholesterol to levels below then current guideline recommendations for high risk patients could further benefit these patients irrespective of their baseline LDL-cholesterol levels. In fact, the real magnitude of benefit from statins may be even higher than reported considering that compliance was 85% in the statin arm, and 17% of placebo group were using non-study statins.

Along with HOPE (page 26), HPS was another definitive trial to refute the benefits of vitamins in vascular disease.

# PROVE-IT-TIMI 22

Intensive versus Moderate Lipid Lowering with Statins after Acute Coronary Syndromes.
Pravastatin or Atorvastatin Evaluation and Infection Therapy – Thrombolysis in Myocardial Infarction 22 Study.
*New England Journal of Medicine* 2004;350:1495-1504.

## Study Question
Does aggressive lipid lowering to levels below that are recommended by the NCEP-ATP III Guidelines[16] further reduce major adverse cardiac events in patients presenting with ACS?

## Methods
Double blind, randomized controlled trial which enrolled 4,162 patients presenting with an ACS.
Patients were randomized to pravastatin 40mg or atorvastatin 80mg daily.
Primary endpoint: a composite of death, MI, UA requiring re-hospitalization, revascularization (>30 days after randomization), and stroke.
Follow up was 18-36 months (mean of 24).

## Results
At the end of the trial, median LDL levels in the atorvastatin arm were significantly lower than in the pravastatin group (1.6 mmol/L vs. 2.46 mmol/L $p<0.001$)

*Atorvastatin vs. Pravastatin*:

| | | | |
|---|---|---|---|
| Primary endpoint: | 22.4% vs. 26.3% | RRR 16% | (p=0.005) |
| Unstable angina: | 3.8% vs. 5.1% | RRR 29% | (p=0.02) |
| Revascularization: | 16.3% vs. 18.8% | RRR 14% | (p=0.04) |
| Death or MI: | 8.3% vs. 10% | RRR 18% | (p=0.06) |
| Death: | 2.2% vs. 3.2% | RRR 28% | (p=0.07) |
| Stroke: | 1.0% vs. 1.0% | NS | |

The benefit of atorvastatin was consistent across all pre-specified subgroups and was seen as early as 30 days into the study.
Rates of drug discontinuation were not different between groups.

### Adverse events
*Atorvastatin vs. Pravastatin:*

| | | |
|---|---|---|
| LE elevations (>3x ULN): | 1.1% vs. 3.3% | (p<0.001) |
| Myalgia or CK elevation: | 2.7% vs. 3.3% | (p=0.23) |
| Rhabdomyolysis: | none in either group. | |

## Conclusion

ACS patients treated with the high-dose atorvastatin received greater protection against death or major cardiovascular events than those treated with pravastatin 40mg daily.

## Perspective

This study (and the similarly designed but much smaller angiographic study, REVERSAL[17]) prompted a revision of the prevailing ACC/AHA Guidelines. The new version stated that in patients with an ACS it is reasonable to aggressively lower LDL levels to 1.8 mmol/L or less (i.e., the mean on-treatment LDL cholesterol level for the atorvastatin group).

The results of this study are remarkable in that the benefit of atorvastatin was seen despite the fact that the pravastatin group achieved the Guideline-recommended targets of LDL cholesterol (<2.5 mmol/L). In addition, the benefit of atorvastatin was demonstrated over and above the comprehensive secondary prevention and early invasive strategy that both groups received.

It is interesting to note that a subgroup analysis of this study showed that patients in the pravastatin group who achieved an LDL-cholesterol level of 1.6 mmol/L or less had the same benefits as the patients in the atorvastatin group. This suggests that the observed benefits are due to aggressive LDL-cholesterol lowering rather than being drug specific.

A similar trial, TNT[18] enrolled 10,001 patients with stable CHD and LDL-C levels of <3.4 mmol/L already tolerating 10mg of atorvastatin. These patients were randomized to continue with 10mg or to receive 80mg of atorvastatin daily for 5 years. The latter group had a 22% RRR of CV death, nonfatal MI, resuscitation after cardiac arrest, or stroke (p<0.001). Overall mortality was not reduced.

One of the most frequent criticisms of recent statin-trials, like TNT and PROVE-IT, is that there is no statistically significant benefit in overall mortality. However, since previous studies such as the 4S (page 32), adequately powered to detect differences in mortality, have clearly demonstrated the mortality benefits associated with the use of statins randomizing patients with CVD to placebo is no longer ethical. Therefore, currently patients can only be involved in studies that treat both arms somewhat differently. In the 4S study that showed a mortality benefit, the LDL-C difference between the two arms was 38%, in PROVE-IT the difference was only about 30%, which still translated into a trend towards improved mortality. In TNT the LDL-difference of 22% in the two treatment arms resulted in a morbidity benefit only and in other studies like the ALLHAT-LLT[19], where the control arm was relatively aggressively treated the difference was only 9%, and therefore, no benefit was seen at all. If we still wanted to carry out trials that are powered to detect a mortality difference we would need mega trials with sample sizes in the range of 30,000-50,000, which is very challenging if at all possible. Thus, if we conduct trials in which the treatment arms are treated differently, but still in an ethically acceptable manner, comparative studies are likely only to demonstrate morbidity reductions. Furthermore, as evidenced by TNT, COURAGE (page 21), TRANSCEND (page 29) and PEACE[14], current therapy results in such low mortality in both treatment and control groups that any further treatment benefit may be challenging to demonstrate.

16. NCEP ATP III Guidelines: *Circulation* 2002;106:3143-3421.
17. REVERSAL: *JAMA* 2004;291:1071-80.
18. TNT: *N Engl J Med* 2005;352:1425-1435.
19. ALLHAT-LLT: *JAMA* 2002;288:2998-3007.

# Hypertension

## ALLHAT

Major Outcomes in High-Risk Hypertensive Patients Randomized to Angiotensin-converting Enzyme Inhibitor or Calcium Channel Blocker vs. Diuretic.
The Antihypertensive and Lipid-Lowering Treatment to Prevent Heart Attack Trial.
*JAMA* 2002;288:2981-2997.

### Study Question
What is the best pharmacologic regimen for the treatment of high blood pressure? What are the comparative benefits of different treatment regimens?

### Methods
Double blind randomized controlled trial of 33,357 adults over the age of 55 years with HTN and one other CV risk factor.
Patients were randomized to one of three possible antihypertensives: ACE inhibitor (lisinopril) or CCB (amlodipine) or diuretic (chlorthalidone). Open label drugs (atenolol or reserpine or clonidine or hydralazine) could be added if patient were not at BP target (140/90 mmHg).
Mean follow up was 4.9 years.

### Results
Blood pressure was significantly higher in the lisinopril (2 mmHg) and the amlodipine (0.8 mmHg) groups compared to chlorthalidone.
There was no difference between the 3 groups for the primary outcome (CV death or MI) or all cause mortality.

**Primary outcome: CV death or nonfatal MI**
*Lisinopril vs. Chlorthalidone:* 11.4% vs. 11.5%   RR 0.99 (95% CI 0.91-1.08)
*Amlodipine vs. Chlorthalidone:* 11.3% vs. 11.5%   RR 0.98 (95% CI 0.90-1.07)

**Secondary outcomes:**
*Lisinopril vs. Chlorthalidone:*
CV morbidity: 33.3% vs. 30.9%   RR 1.10 (95% CI 1.05-1.16)
Stroke:       6.3% vs. 5.6%     RR 1.15 (95% CI 1.02-1.30)
HF:           8.7% vs. 7.7%     RR 1.19 (95% CI 1.07-1.31)

*Amlodipine vs. Chlorthalidone:*
HF:           10.2% vs. 7.7%    RR 1.38 (95% CI 1.25-1.52)

*Chlorthalidone vs. lisinopril:*
New diabetes:      11.6% vs. 8.1%   (p<0.001)
New dyslipidemia: 14.4% vs. 12.8%   (p<0.001)

## Conclusion

The thiazide diuretic chlorthalidone is as good as other, more expensive, antihypertensives with respect to preventing cardiovascular outcomes. No excess in cardiovascular events was seen in the chlorthalidone group despite an excess of new diabetes and increase in lipid profiles.

## Perspective

Initial antihypertensive studies showed important benefits of pharmacologic antihypertensive treatment compared to placebo. ALLHAT was the largest trial to address the question of which medications or combinations are better for the treatment of hypertension. The results of ALLHAT suggest that chlorthalidone strikes the best balance of efficacy and economy. Many experts believe that these results can be extrapolated to other thiazide diuretics such as hydrochlorothiazide. However, metabolic side effects, such as higher rates of new diabetes and new dyslipidemia, have tempered the enthusiasm to widely use them as first-line therapy. Nevertheless, thiazides remain very popular as second- or third-line agents in combination with other drugs, such as ACE inhibitors, ARBs and calcium channel blockers.

ALLHAT was criticized because it enrolled 35% African Americans, who respond to diuretics and CCBs better than to ACE inhibitors. Furthermore, drugs of the primary randomization could not be combined, and this restriction would not be consistent with current practice. Most patients with HTN are unable to achieve BP targets on one drug. Therefore, it is rather meaningless to compare individual medications to each other.

Similar trials[20-26] did not find major differences in hard outcomes between drug classes with the possible exception of the recent ACCOMPLISH trial.[27] This study found the CCB/ACE-I combination to be better than the HCTZ/ACE-I combination despite similar blood pressure reduction on both arms.

The current evidence-based opinion is that some antihypertensive drugs may be better suited for certain individuals, but the most important goal remains to diagnose HTN and to significantly decrease BP in hypertensive patients.

20. LIFE: *Lancet* 2002;359:995-1003.
21. AASK: *JAMA* 2001;285:2719-28 and 2002;288:2421-31.
22. INVEST: *JAMA* 2003;290:2805-16.
23. INSIGHT: *Lancet* 2000;356:366-72.
24. SCOPE: *J Hypertension* 2003;21:875-86.
25. VALUE: *Lancet* 2004;363:2022-2031 and pages 2049-2051.
26. ASCOT: *Lancet* 2005;366:895-906.
27. ACCOMPLISH: *N Engl J Med* 2008;359:2417-28.

# Heart Failure/LV Dysfunction

## SOLVD

Studies of Left Ventricular Dysfunction
*New England Journal of Medicine* 1991;325:293-302, and
*New England Journal of Medicine* 1992;327:685-691.

### Study Question
Does enalapril reduce mortality and morbidity in patients with low ejection fraction with or without heart failure?

### Methods
Double blind randomized controlled trial testing the effects of enalapril in the treatment and prevention of heart failure.

All 5,025 patients enrolled in the trial had LV systolic dysfunction (EF ≤35%). Patients were then stratified into two populations according to whether or not they had symptomatic heart failure. Patients with symptomatic heart failure formed the group which tested the enalapril treatment hypothesis and those without heart failure tested the enalapril prevention hypothesis.

Treatment arm: 2,569 patients, 90% NYHA II-III; follow up: 3.4 years.

Prevention arm: 4,228 patients; follow up of 37.4 months.

All patients were randomized to enalapril 2.5-5mg BID increased to 5-10mg BID in 2 weeks or placebo.

### Results
**Treatment trial:** Final mean dose of enalapril: 16.6mg.

*Enalapril vs. Placebo:*

| | | | |
|---|---|---|---|
| Mortality: | 35.2% vs. 39.7% | RRR 16% | (p=0.0036) |
| Death or HF admission: | 47.7% vs. 57.3% | RRR 26% | (p<0.0001) |

**Prevention trial:**

*Enalapril vs. Placebo:*

| | | | |
|---|---|---|---|
| Total mortality: | 14.8% vs. 15.8% | RRR 8% | (p=0.3) |
| CV mortality: | 12.6% vs. 14.1% | RRR 12% | (p=0.12) |
| Death and new HF: | 29.8% vs. 38.6% | RRR 29% | (p<0.001) |

### Conclusion
Enalapril significantly reduced mortality in patients with chronic heart failure and LV dysfunction.

In patients with asymptomatic left ventricular dysfunction there was only a trend towards reduced CV mortality but the combined endpoint of death and hospitalization for HF was significantly reduced by enalapril.

## Perspective

A series of similar studies conducted with different ACE inhibitors (SAVE, AIRE, TRACE, V-HeFT II, CONSENSUS[28-32] etc.) showed very similar results. ACE inhibitors significantly decreased mortality and heart failure admissions in patients with chronic heart failure as well as in post-MI LVD with or without HF. Therefore, ACE inhibitors became first-line therapy and remain the mainstay of treatment in systolic heart failure and in asymptomatic LV dysfunction both post MI as well as in non-ischemic cardiomyopathy, although there is limited data in this group.

28. SAVE: *N Engl J Med* 1992;327:669-677.
29. AIRE: *Lancet* 1993;342:821-8.
30. TRACE: *N Engl J Med* 1995;333:1670-6.
31. V-HeFT II: *N Engl J Med* 1991;325:303-10.
32. CONSENSUS: *N Engl J Med* 1987;316:1429-35.

# DIG

The Effect of Digoxin on Mortality and Morbidity in Patients with Heart Failure. The Digitalis Investigation Group.
*New England Journal of Medicine* 1997;336:525-533.

## Study Question
Does digoxin improve mortality and morbidity in heart failure?

## Methods
Double blind RCT in which patients with HF and LVEF $\leq$45% were randomized to digoxin (median dose, 0.25mg daily) or placebo in addition to diuretics and ACE inhibitors (average follow up, 37 months). In a secondary trial of patients with heart failure and EF>45%, 988 patients were randomly assigned to digoxin or placebo. Only patients in normal sinus rhythm were randomized.

## Results
*Digoxin vs. Placebo*:

| | | |
|---|---|---|
| Overall mortality: | 34.8% vs. 35.1% | (p=0.80) |
| Death due to worsening HF: | 11.6% vs. 13.2% | (RRR 12%, p=0.06) |
| Hospitalization for worsening HF: | 26.8% vs. 34.7 % | (RRR 28%, p<0.001) |

Subgroup analysis demonstrated that patients with worse heart failure received the most benefit from digoxin.

### Adverse events
*Digoxin vs. Placebo:*

| | | |
|---|---|---|
| VT or cardiac arrest: | 4.2% vs. 4.3% | (p=NS) |

## Conclusion
Digoxin did not reduce overall mortality, but it reduced the rate of hospitalization for worsening HF.

## Perspective
Over the past 15 years there has been substantial enthusiasm for the use of intravenous and oral positive inotropes to improve symptoms and outcomes in patients with systolic heart failure. To date almost all studies of potent inotropes have demonstrated improved symptoms at the cost of increased complications, including mortality.

While the DIG study failed to demonstrate a mortality benefit it did achieve important quality of life endpoints such as improved HF symptoms and reduced hospital admissions. In the current era of evidence based practice, any medical therapy must show a reduction in 'hard' cardiovascular endpoints to gain widespread endorsement. That being said, digoxin remains useful in patients with ongoing symptoms of congestion.

# CHARM

Candesartan in Heart Failure Assessment of Reduction in Mortality and Morbidity.
CHARM-Overall: *Lancet* 2003;362:759-766.
CHARM-Added: *Lancet* 2003;362:767-771.
CHARM-Alternative: *Lancet* 2003;362:772-776.
CHARM-Preserved: *Lancet* 2003;362:777-781.

## Study Question

1) Does the angiotensin II receptor antagonist candesartan improve heart failure and mortality in patients with heart failure who are already on ACE inhibitors?
2) Can ACE-intolerant heart failure patients tolerate candesartan and does it improve on their cardiovascular outcomes?
3) Does candesartan improve cardiovascular outcomes of patients with heart failure and preserved LV systolic function?

## Methods

**CHARM-Overall** was a double blind randomized controlled trial of 7,601 patients with chronic heart failure. All enrolled patients were randomized to candesartan or placebo. Three component studies were carried out simultaneously that stratified patients according to:

1. Concomitant use of ACE inhibitor    (**CHARM-Added**, n = 2,548)
2. Intolerance to ACE inhibitor    (**CHARM-Alternative**, n = 2,028)
3. Preserved ejection fraction    (**CHARM-Preserved**, n = 3,023)

Follow up was at least 2 years.
The primary endpoint of the main trial was all-cause mortality.
The primary endpoint for each sub-study was CV death or hospital admission for CHF.

## Results

### CHARM – Overall

*Candesartan vs. Placebo:*
Death:       23% vs. 25%     RR 0.91 (95% CI 0.83-1.00, p=0.055)
CV death:      18% vs. 20%     RR 0.88 (95% CI 0.79-0.97, p=0.012)
Admissions for CHF: 20% vs. 24%    (p<0.0001)

More patients discontinued candesartan than placebo because of renal dysfunction, hypotension and hyperkalaemia.

## CHARM-Added

*Candesartan vs. Placebo:*

CV death/HF hospitalization:

       37.9% vs. 42.3%     RR 0.85 (95% CI 0.75-0.96, p=0.011)

CV death:

       23.7% vs. 27.3%     RR 0.84 (95% CI 0.72-0.98, p=0.029)

Admissions for CHF:

       24.2% vs. 28.0%     RR 0.83 (95% CI 0.71-0.96, p=0.01)

Similar results in all predefined subgroups, including patients also receiving baseline beta blocker treatment.

## CHARM-Alternative

*Candesartan vs. Placebo:*

CV death/HF hospitalization:

       33% vs. 40%     RR 0.77 (95% CI 0.67-0.89, p=0.0004)

CV death:

       21.6% vs. 24.8%     RR 0.85 (95% CI 0.71-1.02, p=0.072)

HF hospitalization:

       20.4% vs. 28.2%     RR 0.68 (95% CI 0.57-0.81, p<0.0001)

Study-drug discontinuation rates were similar to placebo.

## CHARM-Preserved

*Candesartan vs. Placebo:*

CV death/HF hospitalization:

       22% vs. 24.3%     RR 0.89 (95% CI 0.77-1.03, p=0.118)

CV death:

       11.2% vs. 11.3%     RR 0.99 (95% CI 0.80-1.22, p=NS)

Admissions for CHF:

       15.9% vs. 18.3%     RR 0.85 (95% CI 0.72-1.01, p=0.072)

## Conclusion

Candesartan significantly reduced the combined endpoint of CV death and hospital admissions for HF in the overall CHARM population, and it was especially effective in patients with decreased EF. The addition of candesartan to an ACE inhibitor led to a reduction in the combined endpoint in patients with CHF and reduced LVEF. Candesartan prevented HF admissions in patients with HF irrespective of LVEF. The drug was generally well tolerated.

## Perspective

CHARM was the largest study to date to assess the efficacy and safety of an angiotensin-receptor blocker (ARB) in chronic HF. However, the results of the CHARM-Overall program are difficult to interpret as CHARM-Overall consists of three trials with three distinct HF patient populations.

CHARM-Added demonstrated a reduction of the combined endpoint of mortality and HF admission with candesartan. However, clinical application of this combination has been hampered by the lack of consistently positive results of other ARB-studies, like Val-HeFT[33] and VALIANT[15] that did not show similarly impressive improvement with the combination of ACE-inhibitors and another ARB, valsartan. After the similarly discouraging results of the combination of telmisartan and ramipril seen in ONTARGET (page 29) Val-HeFT and CHARM remained the only large studies showing some benefits of this combination. Side-effects such as hyperkalemia have been significantly more prevalent due to the combination in all of the above studies.

The issue of hyperkalemia should not be underestimated in light of the impressive results of the RALES study (see page 47) which demonstrated mortality benefit of spironolactone in addition to ACE inhibition in heart failure patients. The benefit of spironolactone was achieved at the expense of slight increases in potassium levels. Given that many heart failure patients will already be on spironolactone and ACE inhibitor, the addition of ARB requires vigilant electrolyte monitoring.

Based on a retrospective analysis, the Val-HeFT Study[33] suggested that the triple combination of an ACE-inhibitor, an ARB and a beta-blocker might have detrimental effects. CHARM-Added refuted this concern.

CHARM-Alternative confirmed that candesartan is both safe and effective in ACE-intolerant patients even if they had ACE-induced angioedema.

Although the CHARM-Preserved arm did not yield a significant mortality benefit it is still the first trial to show that an ARB is effective in patients with heart failure and normal left ventricular function.

33. Val-HeFT: *N Engl J Med* 2001;345:1667-75.

# RALES

Randomized Aldactone Evaluation Study.
*New England Journal of Medicine* 1999;341:709-717.

## Study Question

Does aldactone reduce mortality in patients with advanced heart failure who are already on standard medical therapy including ACE inhibitors?

## Methods

Double blind randomized controlled trial of 1,663 patients with NYHA II-IV HF and LVEF $\leq 35\%$.

Patients randomized to spironolactone 25mg daily or placebo.

Primary endpoint: death from all causes.

## Results

The trial was discontinued early, at 24 months, due to a clear benefit of spironolactone.

*Aldactone vs. Placebo:*

All cause mortality: 34.5% vs. 45.9%    RR 0.70 (95% CI 0.60-0.82, p<0.001)

Death due to HF:    15.5% vs. 22.5%    RR 0.64 (95% CI 0.51-0.80, p<0.001)

Sudden death:      10.0 % vs. 13.1%    RR 0.71 (95% CI 0.54-0.95, p=0.02)

HF hospitalizations:

215 episodes vs. 300 episodes    RR 0.65 (95% CI 0.54-0.77, p<0.001)

**Adverse events**

*Aldactone vs. Placebo:*

Gynecomastia or breast pain in men: 10% vs. 1% (p<0.001)

Hyperkalemia was rare in both groups.

## Conclusion

The aldosterone receptor-blocker spironolactone, in addition to standard therapy, substantially reduced the risk of morbidity and mortality among patients with severe systolic HF.

## Perspective

Rarely in the scientific community has a single study affected practice and guidelines without confirmatory work and replication of the results. With the RALES study, spironolactone therapy became widely accepted and implemented with little hesitation because the trial showed an impressive mortality reduction as well as significant improvement in all the other cardiac endpoints. In addition, spironolactone is inexpensive and does not have a significant hypotensive effect.

The background heart failure therapy among RALES patients was up to then current standards with over 90% of patients receiving an ACE inhibitor, 100% a loop diuretic and 75% digoxin. Only 10% of the patients were on a beta blocker. However, beta blockers exert their beneficial effects via a different mechanism.

The most significant concerns that have arisen from the "real world application" of spironolactone in the treatment of severe heart failure stem from the significantly increased incidence of hyperkalemia and worsening renal function.

A new aldosterone antagonist, eplerenone has also been tested in both the post-AMI[34] and the NYHA Class II heart failure[35] setting. Both trials found this agent to significantly decrease morbidity and mortality, therefore eplerenone may be a suitable alternative for such patients especially if they are intolerant of spironolactone due to gynecomastia.

34. EPHESUS: *N Engl J Med* 2003;348:1309-21.
35. EMPHASIS-HF: *N Engl J Med* 2011;364:11-21.

# MERIT-HF

Effect of Metoprolol CR/XL in Chronic Heart Failure: Metoprolol CR/XL
Randomized Intervention Trial in Congestive Heart Failure.
*Lancet* 1999;353:2001-2007.

## Study Question

Does metoprolol therapy reduce mortality in patients with systolic heart failure
due to ischemic cardiomyopathy?

## Methods

Double blind RCT of 3,991 adults, aged 40-80 years with HF (LVEF <40%)
secondary to IHD. Non-ischemic cardiomyopathy was excluded.
Patients were randomized to metoprolol CR/XL (target dose 200mg/day) vs.
placebo. Administration of metoprolol started at 12.5mg or 25mg/d and
doubled every 2 weeks until the target or the maximum tolerated dose was
achieved.

## Results

The study was stopped early because of significant mortality benefit with
metoprolol. Mean follow up was one year.
Mean daily dose of the study drug was 159mg at the end of the trial.
90% of patients were also on ACE inhibitors and diuretics.

*Metoprolol vs. Placebo:*
All cause annual mortality:

|  |  |  |
|---|---|---|
|  | 7.2% vs. 11% | RR 0.66 (95% CI 0.53–0.81, p=0.00009) |
| CV death: |  | RR 0.62 (95% CI 0.50–0.78, p=0.00003) |
| Sudden cardiac death: |  |  |
|  | 4% vs. 6.7% | RR 0.59 (95% CI 0.45–0.78, p=0.0002) |
| Death from HF: | 1.5% vs. 2.9% | RR 0.51 (95% CI 0.33–0.79, p=0.0023). |

## Conclusion

There is a highly significant mortality benefit with metoprolol treatment in
patients with heart failure secondary to ischemic cardiomyopathy.

## Perspective

For many years the use of negative chronotropic and inotropic agents such as a
beta blocker in heart failure was considered to be absolutely contraindicated.
Further understanding of the pathophysiological mechanism of the negative
feedback spiral with the body's own compensation leading to progressive
congestion and worsening heart failure allowed expansion of therapeutic
options to include agents such as beta blockers.

MERIT-HF was the first moderate sized trial to demonstrate a mortality benefit of beta blockers in ischemic heart failure in patients with an EF <40%. This work was followed up by a host of trials (CIBIS II, COPERNICUS, COMET[36-38] etc.) in both ischemic and non-ischemic HF patient populations that have solidified the use of beta blockers in all patients with systolic heart failure. It is important to recognize that beta blocker therapy should be initiated once patients have achieved clinical stability with other appropriate heart failure medications and the dose should be carefully titrated.

36. CIBIS II: *Lancet* 1999;353:9-13.
37. COPERNICUS: *N Engl J Med* 2001;344:1651-8.
38. COMET: *Lancet* 2003;362:7-13.

# Heart Failure/LV Dysfunction/Arrhythmias

## MADIT-II

Prophylactic Implantation of a Defibrillator in Patients with Myocardial Infarction and Reduced Ejection Fraction.
The Multicenter Automatic Defibrillator Implantation Trial II Investigators.
*New England Journal of Medicine* 2002;346:877-883.

### Study Question
Does ICD implantation improve mortality in patients who have severe LV dysfunction following an AMI but no history of ventricular arrhythmias?

### Methods
Randomized controlled trial designed to evaluate the effect of an implantable defibrillator on survival in 1,232 adults with IHD and EF<30%.
(Excluded: NYHA IV, active CHF, MI within 1 month, or revascularization within 3 months).
Open label 3:2 randomization to Automated Implantable Cardiac Defibrillator (AICD) implantation versus medical therapy.
Average follow up 20 months.

### Results
Patients in both groups were generally on good therapy for IHD and HF (67% on ACE-I, 70% on beta blocker, 67% on statins).
Average LV ejection fraction: 23%.

*AICD vs. Medical Therapy*
Overall mortality: 14.2% vs. 19.8%    RR 0.69 (95% CI 0.51-0.93, p=0.016)
The mortality benefit was only seen after 9 months of AICD implantation.

**Subgroup analysis**
Benefit only if QRS >150msec.

**Adverse events of AICD**
Lead problems: 1.8%.
Infections: 0.7%.
Development of HF (AICD vs. medical therapy): 19.9% vs. 14.9% (p=0.09).

### Conclusion
AICD implantation confers significant mortality benefit in patients with a prior MI and advanced LV dysfunction.

## Perspective

This was the first large trial to show mortality benefit of ICD therapy in patients identified purely by LVEF, QRS width, and functional class. The mortality benefit was similar no matter how long after the index myocardial infarction the ICD was implanted.

There was a non-significant trend to greater heart failure admissions in the AICD group compared to the medical therapy group. The authors propose that by preventing sudden cardiac death, patients survive longer and consequently develop more complications related to their heart failure. In addition, the effects of repeated shocks and chronic ventricular pacing on heart function are not well understood.

Cost-effectiveness remains a problem due to the high cost and limited lifespan of the AICD device. In more recent studies, such as the SCD-HeFT[39], a less expensive, single lead "shock only" ICD was used and that may turn out to be more cost effective.

The effect of additional device therapy (biventricular pacing also known as cardiac resynchronization or CRT) was tested in the RAFT study[40]. Nearly 1800 patients with systolic heart failure and a wide QRS on ECG received ICD implantation and then were randomized to additional CRT. The addition of CRT to an ICD reduced mortality as well as hospitalization for heart failure although this benefit was accompanied by more adverse events particularly around the time of device implantation.

39. SCD-HeFT: *N Engl J Med* 2005;352:225-37.
40. RAFT: *N Engl J Med* 2010;363:2385-95.

# Arrhythmias Including Atrial Fibrillation

## CAST

Cardiac Arrhythmia Suppression Trial.
*New England Journal of Medicine* 1989;321:406-412.

### Study Question
Does suppressing ventricular ectopy with class I antiarrhythmic medications improve mortality in patients post myocardial infarction?

### Method
Double blind randomized controlled trial of 2,309 patients with asymptomatic or mildly symptomatic ventricular arrhythmia after myocardial infarction. Patients were randomized to receive one of three Class I antiarrhythmic agents: encainide, flecainide, or moricizine or placebo.

75% had initial suppression of ventricular ectopy demonstrated by Holter monitor and then were randomized to receive active drug or placebo. Average follow up was 10 months.

### Results
This trial was stopped early due to an excess mortality in the treatment arms.

*Encanide or Flecanide vs. Placebo:*

Death from arrhythmia: 4.5% vs. 1.2%   RR 3.6   (95% CI 1.7-8.5)
Total mortality:      7.7% vs. 3.0%   RR 2.5   (95% CI 1.6-4.5)

### Conclusion
Encainide and flecainide both increased mortality and therefore should not be used in the treatment of patients with asymptomatic or minimally symptomatic ventricular arrhythmia after MI, even though these drugs may be effective initially in suppressing ventricular arrhythmia.

### Perspective
Scientific rigour requires careful interrogation of associations of clinical phenomena in contrast to cause and effect relationships. It had been well established that following acute myocardial infarction, complex ventricular arrhythmias were associated with worse outcomes, including arrhythmic death. Anti-arrhythmic agents were shown to suppress these dysrhythmias and therefore it was believed that these agents would prevent arrhythmic death. The CAST trial provided a very important warning that anti-arrhythmic drugs may increase mortality and therefore their safety must be tested in other patient populations as well. This trial was the first of a series of studies that led physicians to use anti-arrhythmic medications less frequently, especially in acute myocardial infarction, but also across a broad spectrum of cardiovascular disease.

# RE-LY

Dabigatran versus Warfarin in Patients with Atrial fibrillation
*New England Journal of Medicine 2009;361:1139-1151.*

## Study Question
Does Dabigatran prevent the thromboembolic complications of atrial fibrillation as well as warfarin?

## Methods
Multicenter trial of 18,113 patients with atrial fibrillation randomized to twice-daily Dabigatran (110mg or 150mg) or dose adjusted Warfarin. Patients were followed for 2 years for the primary end point of stroke or systemic embolization.

## Results
Complete follow-up was obtained and 99.9% of patients for a median time of two years.
The mean $CHADS_2$ score for study participants was 2.1.

**Primary outcome (stroke or systemic embolization):**

| | | |
|---|---|---|
| Warfarin: | 1.7%/year | |
| Dabigatran 110 mg BID: | 1.5%/year | p=0.001 vs. warfarin |
| Dabigatran 150 mg BID: | 1.1%/year | p=0.001 vs. warfarin |

**Annualized Adverse Events (warfarin vs. Dabigatran 110 mg BID vs. Dabigatran 150 mg BID)**

| | | |
|---|---|---|
| Mortality: | 4.2% vs. 3.8% vs. 3.6% | (p = NS vs. warfarin) |
| Myocardial infarction: | 0.5% vs. 0.7% vs. 0.7% | (p < 0.05 for warfarin vs. dabigatran 150mg) |
| Hemorrhagic stroke: | 0.38% vs. 0.12% 0.10% | (p< 0.001 vs. warfarin) |
| Major bleeding: | 3.4% vs. 2.7% vs. 3.1% | (p = 0.003 warfarin vs. dabigatran 110mg) |

## Conclusion
Dabigatran at a dose of 110mg or 150mg twice daily is a safe and effective alternative to Warfarin for the prevention of stroke and systemic embolization in patients with atrial fibrillation.

## Perspective

For decades warfarin has been the only oral anticoagulant that was safe and effective to prevent thromboembolic complications of atrial fibrillation for patients with moderate to high stroke risk.[41] The effective use of warfarin is complicated by its interactions with food and a multitude of medications. These challenges result either in under anticoagulation with resultant stroke risk or over anticoagulation resulting in major bleeding episodes. Novel oral anticoagulants such as Dabigatran and Apixaban* have promise to eliminate our reliance on warfarin. Dabigatran is a direct, competitive inhibitor of thrombin that does not require regular monitoring. Both doses of dabigatran were non-inferior to warfarin whereas the 150 mg dose was superior to warfarin in the prevention of thromboembolic complications of atrial fibrillation with no additional increase in bleeding risk. It's important to note that achievement of target INR in a carefully monitored clinical trial environment often far exceeds that achieved in the community. This suggests that the relative advantage of dabigatran over warfarin would be predicted to be even greater when compared to 'real life' warfarin use.

In the original RE-LY publication the Dabigatran 150 mg arm had an excess of myocardial infarction compared to warfarin. An update to the RE-LY Trial was approved by the Food and Drug Administration as well as the data and safety monitoring committee and was published in the *New England Journal of Medicine* in November 2010[†]. This update included 81 previously unanalyzed adverse events with the result that there was no longer a statistically significant increase in myocardial infarction in the dabigatran 150 mg arm.

41. Meta-analysis: antithrombotic therapy to prevent stroke in patients who have nonvalvular atrial fibrillation. *Ann Intern Med* 2007;146:857–867.
*Connolly et al *N Engl J Med* 2011;364(9):806-17.
[†]*N Engl J Med* 363;19:1875-6.

# AFFIRM

A Comparison of Rate Control and Rhythm Control in Patients with Atrial Fibrillation.

Atrial Fibrillation Follow up Investigation of Rhythm Management Investigators.
*New England Journal of Medicine* 2002;347:1825-33.

## Study Question

What is the preferred management strategy for patients with atrial fibrillation: rate control or rhythm control?

## Methods

Randomized controlled trial of 4,060 adults over the age of 65 with recurrent atrial fibrillation.

Patients were randomized to rate or rhythm control. Appropriate rate control was defined as HR<80 bpm at rest, and <110 bpm on a 6-minute walk test. Physicians could use their discretion as to the selection of medical regimen. Rhythm control approach included cardioversion if necessary and an anti-arrhythmic of the attending physician's choice. Anticoagulation could be stopped, if patients appeared to be in sinus rhythm for 4-12 weeks.

Mean follow up was 3.5 years.

## Results

Most commonly used anti-arrhythmic medications included amiodarone, sotalol, and propafenone, and 62.5% of patients achieved rhythm control at 5 year follow up.

Most commonly used rate control medications include digoxin, beta blocker, and CCB, and 80% of patients achieved rate control.

*Rate vs. Rhythm:*

| | | |
|---|---|---|
| All cause mortality: | 25.9% vs. 26.7% | (p=0.08) |
| Ischemic stroke*: | 5.5% vs. 7.1% | (p=0.79) |
| Warfarin use: | 90% vs. 70% | |
| Hospitalization: | 73% vs. 80.1% | (p<0.001) |

### Adverse events

*Rate vs. Rhythm:*

| | | |
|---|---|---|
| Torsades de pointes: | 0.2% vs. 0.8% | (p=0.007) |
| Sustained VT: | 0.7% vs. 0.6% | (p=0.44) |

*Two thirds of ischemic strokes in both groups occurred when warfarin was being held or when the patient's INR was sub-therapeutic.

## Conclusion

Management of atrial fibrillation with the rhythm-control strategy offers no survival advantage over the rate-control strategy. Moreover, there are potential advantages, such as a lower risk of adverse drug effects, with the rate-control strategy. Anticoagulation should be continued in this group of high-risk patients regardless of the selected treatment strategy.

## Perspective

The AFFIRM trial results reassured clinicians that aggressive rate-control was a reasonable alternative to rhythm control. Also, antiarrhythmic drugs that were given more often in the rhythm control group have been shown to adversely affect survival especially in patients with IHD, whereas beta blockers, given more often in the rate-control group do not have such an adverse effect and may be even beneficial.

The majority of strokes in both groups occurred when anticoagulation was held or was sub-therapeutic, which underscores the dangers of stopping anticoagulation in patients with paroxysmal atrial fibrillation even if they appear to maintain normal sinus rhythm.

The recently published AF-CHF trial[42] showed very similar results in 1376 patients with chronic HF. Rhythm control was not superior to rate control in any of the outcomes including overall and cardiac mortality, worsening heart failure and stroke.

Despite these considerations practitioners are frequently reminded that a minority of patients cannot tolerate atrial fibrillation well and for these patients rhythm control (with anticoagulation) remains the best option.

42. AF-CHF: *N Engl J Med* 2008;358:2667-2677.

# Hormone Replacement Therapy

## WOMEN'S HEALTH INITIATIVE (WHI)

Risks and Benefits of Estrogen Plus Progestin in Healthy Postmenopausal
Women. Principal Results from the Women's Health Initiative Randomized
Controlled Trial.
*JAMA* 2002;288:321-333.

### Study Question

Is hormone replacement therapy a safe way to reduce cardiovascular events in
postmenopausal women?

### Methods

Double blind randomized controlled trial of 16,608 postmenopausal women (50-
79 years old) with an intact uterus.
Patients were randomized to hormone replacement (0.625mg estrogen + 2.5mg
medroxyprogesterone) or placebo.
Follow up 5.2 years (8.5 planned).
Primary endpoint: nonfatal MI and CHD death.
Primary adverse outcome: invasive breast cancer.

### Results

The trial was stopped early due to excess risk of invasive breast cancer in the
HRT group.
Hazard ratio of main outcomes:

*HRT vs. Placebo:*

| | |
|---|---|
| Total mortality: | 0.98 (95% CI 0.82-1.18) |
| Coronary heart disease: | 1.29 (95% CI 1.02-1.63) |
| Breast cancer: | 1.26 (95% CI 1.00-1.59) |
| Stroke: | 1.41 (95% CI 1.07-1.85) |
| Pulmonary embolism: | 2.13 (95% CI 1.39-3.25) |
| Colorectal cancer: | 0.63 (95% CI 0.43-0.92) |
| Endometrial cancer: | 0.83 (95% CI 0.47-1.47) |
| Hip fracture: | 0.66 (95% CI 0.45-0.98) |

The net effect of estrogen and progestin therapy (per 10,000 person-years) was
5 fewer colorectal cancers and 5 fewer hip fractures at the expense of 7 excess
CHD events, 8 excess strokes, 8 excess pulmonary emboli and 8 more invasive
breast carcinomas.

The adverse cardiovascular outcomes of HRT became evident soon after
randomization whereas the excess risk for breast cancer emerged after about 4
years.

The increased risks associated with HRT were present across all racial/ethnic and age strata.

When the analysis was repeated looking only at patients actually taking HRT (i.e., on-treatment analysis) it showed even higher risks for adverse outcomes than the original intention to treat analysis.

## Conclusion

HRT treatment in postmenopausal women is associated with significant adverse cardiovascular, thromboembolic and malignant events. These data do not support the use of HRT for the prevention of cardiovascular outcomes.

## Perspective

This study put an end to another age-old debate about the usefulness of HRT in preventing cardiovascular events. While there were significant benefits seen regarding hip fractures, almost all the other main outcomes showed increased risks with hormone replacement. In addition, during the time this study was being conducted, new therapies for osteoporosis were identified (i.e., bisphosphonates) that were both safe and effective, rendering HRT obsolete for the indication of osteoporosis prevention. This trial could not distinguish between the effects of estrogen and progestin. The adverse effects of progestin were initially thought to be more important for breast cancer and atherosclerotic diseases than estrogen. However, the final results of the WHI estrogen-only trial confirmed that in 10,739 women who had had a previous hysterectomy, the benefits of estrogen therapy (specifically a reduction in bone fracture) was offset by an increase in stroke and venous thromboembolic events. However, unlike in the main trial, in this patient population there was no increased risk for breast cancer found.[43]

43. WHI Estrogen only Study: *Arch Intern Med* 2006;166:357-65.

# Diabetes and the Heart

## ADVANCE

Effects of a fixed combination of perindopril and indapamide on macrovascular and microvascular outcomes in patients with type 2 diabetes mellitus (the ADVANCE trial): a randomized controlled trial.
*Lancet* 2007;370:829-40.

Intensive blood glucose control and vascular outcomes in patients with type 2 diabetes
*New England Journal of Medicine* 2008;358:2560-72.

### Study Question
Does tight blood pressure and intensive glucose control reduce vascular complications and mortality of Type II diabetes mellitus (DM) in the current era?

### Methods
Randomized controlled trial of 11,140 patients with type II DM, a history of a microvascular or macrovascular complication, or at least one more risk factor. Patients requiring insulin therapy were excluded.

Randomization: perindopril (2mg) and indapamide (0.625mg) or placebo in addition to current treatment. After 3 months the doses were increased to 4mg and 1.25mg, respectively.

The trial had another randomization in a 2x2 factorial design to more or less intensive glucose control which was published separately. Intensive glucose control was achieved if HbA1c dropped to 6.5% or less.

The primary outcome was a composite of microvascular and macrovascular events including death, non-fatal MI, non-fatal stroke, new or worsening nephropathy or retinopathy.
Mean follow-up was 4.3 years.

### Results

BP Control
   *Perindopril plus indapamide vs. placebo:*
   BP reduction (mean baseline 145/81 mmHg): 5.6/2.2 mmHg  ($p < 0.0001$)
   Major micro+macrovascular events:
                      15.5% vs. 16.8%      RR 0.91 (95% CI 0.83–1.0;  p=0.041)

Major micro\*- *or* macrovascular[†] events *separately* showed NS benefits (p=0.16)

Death: 7.3% vs. 8.5% RR 0.86 (95% CI 0.98-0.75; p=0.025)

CV death: 3.8% vs. 4.6% RR 0.82 (95% CI 0.98-0.68; p=0.027)

Coronary events: 8.4% vs. 9.6% RR 0.86 (95% CI 0.98-0.76; p=0.02)

Cerebrovascular events: RR 0.94 p=0.41

Renal events (mainly new albuminuria):RR 0.79 (95% CI 0.85-0.73; p<0.0001)

Visual deterioration: RR 0.95 (95% CI 0.90-1.01; p=0.10)

\*Major microvascular events included new or worsening nephropathy, or retinopathy.

[†]Major macrovascular endpoints included CV death, non-fatal MI or non-fatal stroke.

### Glucose control (intensive vs. not)

Mean HbA1c: 6.5% vs. 7.3% (p<0.008)

Major micro+macrovascular events:

18.1% vs. 20.0% RR 0.90 (95% CI 0.82-0.98; p=0.01)

Major microvascular events: RR 0.86 (95% CI 0.77-0.97; p=0.01)

Major macrovascular events: RR 0.94 (95% CI 0.84-1.06; p=NS)

Death: RR 0.93 (95% CI 0.83-1.06; p=NS)

Renal events: RR 0.79 (95% CI 0.66-0.93; p=0.006)

Visual deterioration: NS

## Conclusion

"Routine administration of a fixed combination of perindopril and indapamide to patients with type 2 diabetes was well tolerated and reduced the risks of major vascular events, including death. Although the confidence limits were wide, the results suggest that over 5 years, one death due to any cause would be averted among every 79 patients assigned active therapy."

Intensive glucose control yielded a modest reduction in major macrovascular and microvascular events, primarily as a consequence of a 21% relative reduction in nephropathy.

## Perspective

The UKPDS studies[44-47] provided the first evidence in the 1980s that tight BP and glucose control may not only be logical and prudent, but that they also decrease the risk of diabetic complications. The magnitude of benefit, however, was not all that impressive likely due to the fact that each individual UKPDS study attempted to control only one risk factor (i.e. diabetes or hypertension) and lipid control was not systematically addressed at all.

The ADVANCE trial studied the same question in a more comprehensive fashion in a more current environment. It assessed the effect of tight glucose control and that of a fixed combination of the long-acting ACE-inhibitor perindopril and the diuretic indapamide versus placebo added to usual care. Unfortunately, the latter arm of the trial became one of more aggressive BP control vs. less aggressive BP control where the placebo arm did not get even close to recommended targets. Furthermore, less than half of these diabetic patients were treated with statins and just over half received antiplatelet therapy. Nevertheless, the benefits, especially the significant reduction in overall and cardiovascular mortality are encouraging.

Intensive glucose control yielded similarly modest benefits. However, the exact benefits versus the risks of aggressive glucose control remain controversial. The ACCORD[48] trial that also tested the effects of tight glucose control found an increased risk of death on the intensive treatment arm that led to the early discontinuation of this study. The increased mortality persisted out to 5 years of follow up despite the fact that aggressive glucose management was discontinued after 3.5 years of follow-up.[49] Interestingly, patients with the lowest HbA1c throughout the study had the lowest mortality and aggressive diabetes management actually reduced the risk of myocardial infarction. Therefore the observed increase in mortality is even more difficult to explain.

A recent analysis proposed that this paradox result was possibly due to the fact that patients whose diabetes was uncontrolled at randomization and could not be improved during the trial had an increased mortality affecting the results on the intensive treatment arm.[50] Until this issue is clarified aggressive blood sugar control to aim for a HbA$_1$C to less than 6% should be avoided.

On balance, the majority of the available evidence supports an aggressive approach to reducing all risk factors in diabetic patients.

44. UKPDS 38: *British Medical Journal* 1998;317:703-713.
45. UKPDS 39: *British Medical Journal* 1998;317:713-720.
46. UKPDS 33: *Lancet* 1998;352:837-853.
47. UKPDS 34: *Lancet* 1998;352:854-865.
48. ACCORD: *N Engl J Med* 2008;358:2545-59.
49. ACCORD: Long-term effects. *N Engl J Med* 2011;364:818-828.
50. ACCORD post hoc analysis: *Diabetes Care* 2010;33:983-90.

# Additional References

1. ISIS-2: *Lancet* 1986;328:57-66.

2. COMMIT-CCS 2 - clopidogrel arm: *Lancet* 2005;366:1607-21.

3. FRISC II: *Lancet* 1999;354:708-15.

4. ESSENCE: *N Engl J Med* 1997;337:447-52.

5. TIMI 11B: *Circulation* 1999;100:1593-1601.

6. ICTUS: *N Engl J Med* 2005;353:1095-1104.

7. ISAR-COOL: *JAMA* 2003;290:1593-9.

8. CURE. *N Engl J Med* 2001;345:494-502.

9. PCI CURE: *Lancet* 2001;358:527-533.

10. INTERHEART: *Lancet* 2004;364:937-952.

11. An INTERHEART Substudy: Parental History and MI Risk Across the World. *J Am Coll Cardiol* 2011;57:619-627.

12. IMAGINE: *Circulation* 2008;117:24-31.

13. EUROPA: *Lancet* 2003;362:782-788.

14. PEACE: *N Engl J Med* 2004;351:2058-68.

15. VALIANT: *N Engl J Med* 2003;349:1893-1906.

16. REVERSAL: *JAMA* 2004;291:1071-80.

17. TNT: *N Engl J Med* 2005;352:1425-1435.

18. NCEP ATP III Lipid Guidelines: *Circulation* 2002;106:3143-3421.

19. ALLHAT-LLT: *JAMA* 2002;288:2998-3007.

20. LIFE: *Lancet* 2002;359:995-1003.

21. AASK: *JAMA* 2001;285:2719-28 and 2002;288:2421-31.

22. INVEST: *JAMA* 2003;290:2805-16.

23. INSIGHT: *Lancet* 2000;356:366-72.

24. SCOPE: *J Hypertension* 2003;21:875-86.

25. VALUE: *Lancet* 2004;363:2022-2031 and pages 2049-2051.

26. ASCOT: *Lancet* 2005;366:895-906.

27. ACCOMPLISH: *N Engl J Med* 2008;359:2417-28.

28. SAVE: *N Engl J Med* 1992;327:669-677.

29. AIRE: *Lancet* 1993;342:821-8.

30. TRACE: *N Engl J Med* 1995;333:1670-6.

31. V-HeFT II: *N Engl J Med* 1991;325:303-10.

32. CONSENSUS: *N Engl J Med* 1987;316:1429-35.

33. Val-HeFT: *N Engl J Med* 2001;345:1667-75.

34. EPHESUS: *N Engl J Med* 2003;348:1309-21.

35. EMPHASIS-HF: *N Engl J Med* 2011;364:11-21.

36. CIBIS II: *Lancet* 1999;353:9-13.

37. COPERNICUS: *N Engl J Med* 2001;344:1651-8.

38. COMET: *Lancet* 2003;362:7-13.

39. SCD-HeFT: *N Engl J Med* 2005;352:225-37.

40. RAFT: *N Engl J Med* 2010;363:2385-95.

41. Meta-analysis: antithrombotic therapy to prevent stroke in patients who have nonvalvular atrial fibrillation. *Ann Intern Med* 2007;146:857–867.

42. AF-CHF: *N Engl J Med* 2008;358:2667-2677.

43. WHI Estrogen only Study: *Arch Intern Med* 2006;166:357-65.

44. UKPDS 38: *British Medical Journal* 1998;317:703-713.

45. UKPDS 39: *British Medical Journal* 1998;317:713-720.

46. UKPDS 33: *Lancet* 1998;352:837-853.

47. UKPDS 34: *Lancet* 1998;352:854-865.

48. ACCORD: *N Engl J Med* 2008;358:2545-59.

49. ACCORD 5-year follow up: Long-term effects. *N Engl J Med* 2011;364:818-828.

50. ACCORD post hoc analysis: *Diabetes Care* 2010;33:983-90.